CURE FOR HIV DISEASE

UNRAVELING THE CURE FOR HIV

Zaackiey Wholist

TABLE OF CONTENT

INTRODUCTION

BRIEF OVERVIEW OF THE HIV/AIDS PANDEMIC

The HIV/AIDS pandemic is a worldwide health crisis that emerged within the overdue twentieth century, due to the human immunodeficiency virus (HIV). The virus ordinarily attacks the immune system, particularly CD4 cells (T cells), which play a important position in the frame's protection in opposition to infections and sicknesses. As the immune device weakens, individuals turn out to be liable to opportunistic infections and certain cancers, main to received immunodeficiency syndrome (AIDS).

Key factors in the review of the HIV/AIDS pandemic consist of:

1. Emergence and Spread:

- The earliest instances of AIDS were pronounced inside the United States in the early Eighties.

- The virus is thought to have originated from simian immunodeficiency virus (SIV) in nonhuman primates and transmitted to human beings in Central Africa, in particular the Democratic Republic of Congo.

2. Global Impact:
   - HIV/AIDS quick spread global, affecting various populations.
   - Sub Saharan Africa has been disproportionately affected, with a high prevalence of HIV infections and AIDS associated deaths.

3. Modes of Transmission:
   - HIV is on the whole transmitted thru unprotected sexual sex, sharing of contaminated needles, and from mother to toddler in the course of childbirth or breastfeeding.
   - Awareness campaigns have emphasized more secure sex practices, needle alternate

applications, and prevention of MOMTOCHILD transmission to reduce new infections.

4. Social and Economic Impact:

- The pandemic has had profound social and economic effects, affecting groups, households, and economies.

- Stigmatization and discrimination in opposition to individuals residing with HIV/AIDS remain substantial demanding situations.

5. Medical Advances:

- The improvement of antiretroviral therapy (ART) has converted HIV/AIDS from a once deadly disorder to a manageable persistent circumstance.

- ART helps suppress the virus, allowing people with HIV to lead more healthy lives and reducing the danger of transmission.

6. Challenges and Ongoing Efforts:

- Despite giant progress, demanding situations persist, consisting of get admission to to treatment, stigma, and the need for a definitive remedy.

- International companies, governments, NGOs, and groups retain to paintings collaboratively to prevent new infections and improve treatment get right of entry to.

THE IMPACT ON INTERNATIONAL FITNESS AND AFFECTED POPULATIONS

The impact of the HIV/AIDS pandemic on global health and affected populations has been profound, encompassing diverse dimensions together with public fitness, social dynamics, and economic stability.

1. Public Health Burden:

- HIV/AIDS has positioned a massive burden on public fitness structures worldwide.

- High prices of infection and the progression to AIDS have strained healthcare infrastructures, especially in areas with restrained assets.

2. Mortality and Morbidity:

- AIDS related illnesses have brought about a tremendous variety of deaths globally, particularly in the absence of effective treatment.

- HIV/AIDS has contributed to expanded morbidity, with individuals going through a better chance of opportunistic infections and sure cancers.

3. Disproportionate Impact on Vulnerable Communities:

- Certain populations, such as men who have intercourse with men, intercourse people, injecting drug users, and transgender people, are disproportionately laid low with HIV/AIDS because of social, economic, and structural elements.

Stigma and discrimination exacerbate vulnerability and avert prevention and treatment efforts.

4. Economic Consequences:

- The financial impact of the pandemic is obvious via lost productivity, improved healthcare expenses, and decreased personnel capability.
- Households tormented by HIV/AIDS may face monetary stress due to medical prices and the loss of income earners.

5. Impact on Children and Families:

- The epidemic has left many children orphaned or vulnerable as mother and father succumb to AIDS related illnesses.
- Families managing HIV/AIDS face social and economic demanding situations, impacting the overall well being of kids.

6. Education and Social Dynamics:

- The pandemic has disrupted education systems, in particular in areas with high infection prices.

- Stigma related to HIV/AIDS can result in social isolation, discrimination, and challenges in getting access to training and employment opportunities.

7. Global Migration and Displacement:

- Migration styles are motivated by way of HIV/AIDS, as individuals can also move searching for higher healthcare, monetary opportunities, or to break out stigma.

- Displacement due to the pandemic can strain social support networks and make contributions to the spread of the virus.

8. International Response and Aid:

- The international network has mobilized assets and released initiatives to cope with HIV/AIDS, such as investment for research, prevention programs, and treatment get right of entry to.

- International corporations, NGOs, and governments collaborate to fight the pandemic, reflecting a commitment to international fitness equity.

CURRENT TREATMENT METHODS AND THEIR BOUNDARIES

As of my final understanding update in January 2022, HIV/AIDS is in most cases managed thru antiretroviral therapy (ART), a mixture of medicinal drugs that concentrate on the virus and sluggish down its replication. It's vital to notice that traits in scientific research may additionally have befell when you consider that then, and remedy guidelines may additionally have advanced.

1. Antiretroviral Therapy (ART):

- ART consists of a mixture of various classes of antiretroviral pills, including nucleoside opposite transcriptase inhibitors (NRTIs), no nucleoside opposite transcriptase inhibitors (NNRTIs), protease inhibitors (PIs), integrate inhibitors (INSTIs), and access/fusion inhibitors. These drugs work by interfering with different stages of the HIV life cycle; preventing the virus from replicating and reducing the viral load in the body.

2. Effectiveness of ART:

- ART has been surprisingly effective in suppressing viral replication, enhancing immune characteristic, and extending the lifespan of people living with HIV.

- When taken constantly and correctly, ART can reduce the viral load to undetectable stages, which no longer most effective benefits the man or woman's health however additionally prevents the sexual transmission of HIV.

3. Challenges and Limitations:

- Adherence Issues: Strict adherence to ART is critical for its effectiveness. Missing doses or irregular medicine schedules can cause the development of drug resistant lines of the virus.

- Side Effects: Some antiretroviral drugs may also purpose aspect results, ranging from mild to extreme. These can encompass nausea, diarrhea, fatigue, and metabolic complications.

- Drug Resistance: Prolonged use of antiretroviral pills can lead to the improvement of drug resistant strains of HIV, proscribing remedy alternatives.

- Access to Treatment: Access to ART varies globally, and some areas face demanding situations in presenting consistent and good sized get right of entry to medicinal drug due to factors together with cost, infrastructure, and healthcare systems.

Adherence Issues: Strict adherence to ART is crucial for its effectiveness. Missing doses or irregular medication schedules can lead to the development of drug resistant strains of the virus.

- Side Effects: Some antiretroviral drugs may cause side effects, ranging from mild to severe. These can include nausea, diarrhea, fatigue, and metabolic complications.

- Drug Resistance: Prolonged use of antiretroviral drugs can lead to the development of drug resistant strains of HIV, limiting treatment options.

- Access to Treatment: Access to ART varies globally, and some regions face challenges in providing consistent and widespread access to medication due to factors such as cost, infrastructure, and healthcare systems.

- HIV in the main goals CD4 T cells, which are imperative to coordinating immune responses against pathogens.
- Progressive depletion of CD4 T cells weakens the immune device's capability to govern HIV and increases susceptibility to opportunistic infections feature

CHAPTER ONE: UNDERSTANDING HIV

THE BASICS OF HIV/AIDS TRANSMISSION AND INFECTION

THE FEATURE OF THE IMMUNE TOOL IN STOPPING THE VIRUS

The immune device performs a crucial position in combating the human immunodeficiency virus (HIV) with the aid of mounting a multifaceted reaction aimed toward controlling viral replication, clearing infected cells, and stopping the progression to acquired immunodeficiency syndrome (AIDS).

1. Innate Immune Response:

- The innate immune device is the body's first line of protection in opposition to pathogens, including viruses like HIV.
- Innate immune cells, which consist of macrophages and dendrites cells, recognize HIV thru sample popularity receptors

(PRRs) and provoke an inflammatory response to restriction viral spread.

- Natural killer (NK) cells play a feature in figuring out and putting off HIV infected cells through CYTOTOXIC mechanisms.

2. Adaptive Immune Response:

- The adaptive immune machine generates unique responses in competition to HIV with the aid of the usage of recognizing viral antigens and mounting targeted immune responses.

- Lymphocytes Produce Antibodies In Opposition To HIV proteins that could neutralize the virus and decorate its clearance through other immune cells.

- CD4 T helper cells orchestrate the adaptive immune response by way of activating one of a kind immune cells and facilitating antibody manufacturing.

- CD8 CYTOTOXIC T lymphocytes (CTLs)
  understand and kill HIV infected cells,
  restricting viral replication and controlling
  the infection.

3. Role of CD4 T Cells:

Of AIDS.

4. HIV Evasion Strategies:

- HIV has advanced numerous mechanisms to
  prevent immune detection and clearance,
  inclusive of:

- Rapid mutation and excessive replication
  costs, leading to immune get away from
  antibody and T cellular reputation.

- Latency and status quo of reservoirs in long
  lived cells, permitting the virus to avoid
  immune surveillance and persist despite
  treatment.

- Modulation of host immune responses and
  immune activation, contributing to chronic
  immune dysfunction and infection.

5. Impact of Chronic Immune Activation:

- Persistent immune activation and infection are hallmarks of HIV infection and contribute to ailment development and immune disorder.

- Chronic immune activation can result in exhaustion of immune cells, DYSREGULATION of cytokine signaling, and tissue damage, contributing to HIV associated complications.

CHAPTER TWO: HISTORICAL PERSPECTIVES

MILESTONES IN HIV RESEARCH AND TREATMENT

Notable breakthroughs and setbacks

Notable breakthroughs and setbacks within the area of HIV/AIDS studies have shaped the trajectory of our know-how, prevention, and remedy of the ailment.

BREAKTHROUGHS:

1. Discovery of HIV (19831984):

   - In 19831984, researchers recognized HIV as the virus accountable for inflicting AIDS, revolutionizing our expertise of the epidemic.

2. Development of Antiretroviral Therapy (ART):

   - The advent of ART inside the mid1990s marked a giant breakthrough, reworking HIV/AIDS from a deadly infection to a manageable persistent condition.

- ART suppresses viral replication, improves immune characteristic, and prolongs the lifespan of individuals residing with HIV.

3. Prevention of Mother to Child Transmission (PMTCT):

- PMTCT packages have been notably a hit in decreasing the transmission of HIV from mother to child at some point of pregnancy, childbirth, and breastfeeding.

- Antiretroviral drugs given to pregnant ladies with HIV and their infants have drastically lowered transmission quotes, main to fewer youngsters born with HIV.

4. PREEXPOSURE Prophylaxis (PREP):

- PREP, a preventive medicinal drug taken through HIV negative people, has been proven to seriously reduce the threat of obtaining HIV thru sexual transmission.

The approval and sizeable availability of PREP had been instrumental in HIV prevention efforts, mainly amongst high risk populations.

5. Advancements in Treatment Options:

- The development of more recent classes of antiretroviral pills, including INTEGRASE inhibitors and long acting formulations, has improved remedy options and advanced adherence.

6. Scientific Progress in Understanding HIV Biology:

- Advances in HIV studies have elucidated key elements of the virus's biology, consisting of its replication cycle, mechanisms of immune evasion, and established order of latent reservoirs.

- This knowledge has informed the development of novel therapeutic strategies, such as gene modifying and immune therapies.

Setbacks:

1. Early Failures in Vaccine Development:
   - Despite many years of studies efforts, the development of a powerful HIV vaccine has been elusive.
   - Several promising vaccine applicants have did not display efficacy in clinical trials, highlighting the challenges of HIV vaccine development.

2. Emergence of Drug Resistance:
   - Prolonged use of antiretroviral pills can lead to the improvement of drug resistant traces of HIV, limiting treatment options and posing challenges for disease control.
   - Drug resistance underscores the importance of adherence to treatment regimens and ongoing surveillance of HIV drug resistance styles.

3. Persistence of HIV Reservoirs:

- HIV can set up latent reservoirs in long lived cells, allowing the virus to persist despite suppressive antiretroviral therapy.
- Eradicating latent reservoirs provides a considerable project in reaching a remedy for HIV/AIDS, as cutting-edge remedies do not goal those reservoirs efficaciously.

4. Stigma and Discrimination:

- Stigma and discrimination continue to be pervasive obstacles to HIV prevention, checking out, and treatment, specifically amongst marginalized and inclined populations.
- Stigma can deter people from in search of HIV related services and make a contribution to social isolation and fitness disparities.

LESSONS LEARNED FROM PAST ATTEMPTS TO FIND A CURE

Past attempts to find a cure for HIV/AIDS have yielded valuable instructions that tell modern research strategies and tactics. Here are a few key classes found out from past efforts:

1. Complexity of HIV Biology:

- HIV is a tremendously mutable virus with complex interactions with the host immune gadget. Early attempts to expand a remedy underestimated the demanding situations posed by way of HIV's potential to avoid immune detection and establish latent reservoirs.

- Lesson: Understanding the tricky biology of HIV is essential for growing powerful remedy techniques. Comprehensive procedures that focus on more than one aspects of the virus's lifecycle are wanted.

2. Importance of Multidisciplinary Collaboration:

- HIV/AIDS studies calls for collaboration across numerous fields, including virology, immunology, genetics, pharmacology, and medical medicine.
- Lesson: Successful therapy research is predicated on interdisciplinary collaboration, bringing collectively scientists, clinicians, public health professionals, and affected communities to deal with the complex challenges of HIV/AIDS.

3. Need for Innovative Approaches:

- Traditional drug based strategies, along with antiretroviral therapy, at the same time as powerful in controlling viral replication, have limitations in attaining a therapy because of the endurance of latent reservoirs.
- Lesson: Innovation is critical for advancing remedy studies. New technology and

approaches, such as gene editing, immunotherapy.

4. Importance of Long Term Follow Up:

- Long term monitoring of individuals living with HIV/AIDS is critical for evaluating the sturdiness and protection of capacity remedy interventions.

- Lesson: Rigorous medical research with long term follow up is important to assess the efficacy, safety, and feasibility of therapy strategies. Ethical concerns, consisting of player consent and confidentiality, should be cautiously addressed.

5. Addressing HIV Stigma and Discrimination:

- Stigma and discrimination associated with HIV/AIDS can pose obstacles to cure studies, avert participation in medical trials, and affect get admission to to healthcare services.

- Lesson: Addressing stigma and discrimination is crucial to a success treatment studies. Community engagement, training, and advocacy efforts can help reduce stigma and sell supportive environments for cure studies and implementation.

6. Importance of Global Collaboration:

- HIV/AIDS is a global fitness project that calls for worldwide collaboration and unity. Past successes in HIV/AIDS studies and remedy had been completed thru partnerships among governments, research institutions, civil society groups, and affected communities.

- Lesson: Global collaboration is important for accelerating progress closer to a cure for HIV/AIDS. Sharing information, sources, and first-class practices throughout borders can decorate the effectiveness and effect of remedy studies efforts.

CHAPTER THREE: THE CUTTINGEDGE SCIENCE

ANTIRETROVIRAL THERAPIES AND THEIR EFFECTIVENESS

Antiretroviral remedy (ART) has revolutionized the treatment of HIV/AIDS, transforming the sickness from a once fatal infection to a viable chronic situation. ART includes a mixture of medications that concentrate on specific degrees of the HIV lifecycle, inhibiting viral replication and allowing the immune gadget to get better.

1. Components of ART:

- ART generally consists of a aggregate of three or more antiretroviral tablets from exclusive training. These training encompass:

- Nucleoside opposite transcriptase inhibitors (NRTIs)

- Non nucleoside opposite transcriptase inhibitors (NNRTIs)

- Protease inhibitors (PIs)

- INTEGRASE inhibitors (INSTIs)

- Entry inhibitors, which include CCR5 antagonists and fusion inhibitors

2. Mechanism of Action:

- Each class of antiretroviral capsules objectives a particular step inside the HIV lifecycle. NRTIs, NNRTIs, and INSTIs inhibit the replication of viral genetic cloth, at the same time as PIs save you the cleavage of viral proteins essential for viral maturation.

- By inhibiting viral replication, ART reduces the viral load inside the body, allowing the immune system to get better and feature more effectively.

3. Effectiveness in Suppressing Viral Replication:

- ART is particularly powerful in suppressing viral replication and decreasing the HIV viral load to undetectable ranges in the blood. An undetectable viral load approach that the quantity of HIV in the blood is just too low to be detected with the aid of trendy laboratory exams.

- Suppression of viral replication enables prevent disease development, preserves immune characteristic, and decreases the chance of opportunistic infections and AIDS related complications.

4. Improvement in Immunological Health:

- ART restores immune feature with the aid of increasing CD4 T mobile counts that are essential for coordinating the body's immune responses.

- With powerful ART, people residing with HIV can experience good sized enhancements in their immune feature, lowering their susceptibility to infections and improving overall fitness effects.

5. Reduction in HIV Transmission Risk:

- Effective ART no longer most effective blessings the character's fitness but also plays a key function in HIV prevention efforts.

- Individuals with undetectable viral masses on ART have a considerably decreased danger of transmitting HIV to their sexual companions, a idea known as "treatment as prevention" (TASP).

6. Challenges and Considerations:

- Adherence to ART is crucial for its effectiveness. Missing doses or inconsistent medicine adherence can cause VIROLOGICAL failure and the improvement of drug resistance.

- ART requires lifelong treatment, and individuals may additionally enjoy aspect consequences, drug interactions, and challenges associated with access, affordability, and stigma.

BREAKTHROUGHS IN IMMUNOTHERAPY AND GENE EDITING TECHNOLOGIES

Breakthroughs in immunotherapy and gene modifying technology have opened new avenues for the remedy and ability therapy of HIV/AIDS.

Immunotherapy Breakthroughs:

AND GENE EDITING TECHNOLOGIES

Breakthroughs in immunotherapy and gene enhancing era have opened new avenues for the remedy and capacity therapy of HIV/AIDS.

Immunotherapy Breakthroughs:

1. Broadly Neutralizing Antibodies (BNABS):

- Broadly neutralizing antibodies are a kind of antibody which could understand and bind to a couple of traces of HIV, targeting conserved areas of the virus's envelope protein.

- BNABS have shown promise in HIV prevention and remedy by neutralizing the virus, blocking its entry into host cells, and improving immune responses.

- Clinical trials have tested the efficacy of BNABS in lowering viral load and delaying viral rebound in individuals residing with HIV.

2. Therapeutic Vaccines:

- Therapeutic vaccines purpose to enhance the immune reaction against HIV, either by stimulating antibody production or activating CYTOTOXIC T cells to target HIV infected cells.

- Various vaccine candidates, which include viral vector vaccines, DNA vaccines, and protein subunit vaccines, are being investigated in medical trials.

- While no healing vaccine has but executed a treatment for HIV/AIDS, a few candidates have proven promise in decreasing viral load or delaying ailment progression.

3. Cell Based Therapies:

- Cell based immune therapies involve modifying immune cells, inclusive of T cells, to decorate their potential to goal and cast off HIV infected cells.

- Chimerical antigen receptor (CAR) T mobile remedy, for instance, includes engineering T cells to explicit receptors that apprehend and bind to HIV infected cells, main to their destruction.

- Early stage medical trials of CAR T cell remedy for HIV/AIDS have shown encouraging results in decreasing viral reservoirs and enhancing immune manipulate of the virus.

Gene Editing Breakthroughs:

1. CRISPR/Ca

- In the context of HIV/AIDS, CRISPR/Cas9 may be used to disrupt viral genes, such as the HIV co receptor

CCR5, crucial for viral entry into host cells.

- Preclinical studies have established the feasibility of using CRISPR/Cas9 to edit immune cells, along with CD4 T cells, to confer resistance to HIV contamination.

2. Gene Therapy Approaches:

- Gene therapy goals to introduce therapeutic genes into target cells to accurate genetic defects or confer resistance to sickness.

- In the context of HIV/AIDS, gene remedy procedures involve enhancing immune cells to decorate their resistance to HIV infection or to target and put off HIV infected cells.

- Clinical trials of gene therapy for HIV/AIDS are underway, exploring strategies which include enhancing stem cells to provide HIV resistant immune cells or enhancing the immune machine's ability to apprehend and cast off HIV infected cells.

3. Gene Silencing Techniques:

- Gene silencing techniques, which include RNA interference (RNAI), purpose to inhibit the expression of particular genes involved in HIV replication.

- Small interfering RNAs (SIRNAS) or brief hairpin RNAs (SHRNAS) may be designed to goal viral genes or host mobile factors crucial for HIV replication.

- Preclinical research has confirmed the effectiveness of RNAIBASED approaches in decreasing viral load and suppressing HIV replication in vitro and in animal fashions.

CHAPTER FOUR: PROMISING APPROACHES

THERAPEUTIC VACCINES AND THEIR POTENTIAL

CRISPRBASED GENE EDITING FOR HIV

CRISPRBASED gene editing has emerged as a promising approach for tackling HIV contamination by using focused on the viral genome or host cell elements concerned in viral replication.

1. Targeting Viral Genome:

- One method involves the usage of CRISPRCas9 to without delay goal and cleaves the HIV genome incorporated into the host cellular's DNA. By disrupting important viral genes, including those encoding viral proteins or regulatory elements, CRISPRCas9 can inhibit viral replication and save you the manufacturing of infectious virus particles.

- Several studies have established the feasibility of the use of CRISPRCas9 to target and disrupt precise regions of the HIV genome, including the lengthy terminal repeat (LTR) or important viral genes like gag, POL, and ENV.

2. Targeting Host Cell Factors:

  - Another method entails targeting host cellular elements that are exploited with the aid of HIV for viral replication. For example, the CC CHEMOKINE receptor kind 5 (CCR5) is a CORECEPTOR used by HIV to enter CD4 T cells. By disrupting the CCR5 gene the usage of CRISPRCas9, researchers can generate HIV resistant immune cells.

  - Clinical trials have proven the potential of CCR5edited immune cells, including CD4 T cells or hematopoietic stem cells, to confer resistance to HIV contamination and reduce viral reservoirs in patients.

3. Enhancing Immune Responses:

- CRISPRBASED processes also can be used to beautify immune responses towards HIV. For example, editing immune cells to explicit chimerical antigen receptors (CARs) that target HIV antigens can decorate their capability to apprehend and do away with HIV infected cells.

- Researchers are exploring techniques to engineer immune cells using CRISPRCas9 to beautify their anti HIV activity, along with improving the production of extensively neutralizing antibodies or boosting the activity of CYTOTO

4. Challenges and Considerations:

- Despite the promise of CRISPRBASED gene enhancing for HIV, numerous challenges continue to be. These include off target outcomes, unintended genetic changes, and the potential for viral escape mutations.

- Delivery of CRISPRCas9 additives to target cells, along with immune cells or stem cells, is any other assignment that needs to be addressed for clinical applications.

- Ethical issues, together with patient consent, protection, and long term outcomes of genetic changes, are essential factors inside the development and implementation of CRISPRBASED cures for HIV.

NANOTECHNOLOGY AND INNOVATIVE DRUG DELIVERY METHODS

Nanotechnology has the ability to revolutionize drug shipping methods for HIV/AIDS treatment with the aid of enhancing the efficacy, safety, and focused delivery of antiretroviral tablets.

1. NANOPARTICLE Based Drug Delivery Systems:

- NANOPARTICLES can function vendors or cars for handing over antiretroviral drugs to goal cells and tissues more correctly.
- NANOPARTICLES can be designed to encapsulate or conjugate with antiretroviral pills, defensive them from degradation and enhancing their balance and bioavailability within the frame.
- Surface modifications of NANOPARTICLES can allow centered delivery to precise cellular kinds or tissues, consisting of HIV infected cells or lymphoid tissues, whilst minimizing off target outcomes.

2. Long Acting Formulations:

- Nanotechnology can be used to expand long acting formulations of antiretroviral drugs that provide sustained launch over a prolonged length, reducing the frequency of dosing and improving patient adherence.

- NANOPARTICLEBASED drug delivery systems, consisting of NANOSUSPENS

4. THERANOSTIC NANOSYSTEMS:

- THERANOSTIC NANOPARTICLES combine therapeutic and diagnostic functionalities, permitting simultaneous drug shipping and tracking of remedy response.

THERANOSTIC NANOSYSTEMS may be used to screen viral load, immune responses, or drug concentrations in real time, imparting valuable insights into remedy efficacy and affected person consequences.

5. Combination Therapy Platforms:

- Nanotechnology enables the code livery of a couple of antiretroviral pills or therapeutic agents in an unmarried NANOPARTICLE platform.

- Combination remedy systems can decorate synergistic effects, triumph over drug resistance, and enhance remedy results through focused on more than one pathways or mechanisms of HIV replication simultaneously.

6. Implantable Devices and Nan sensors:

- Implantable gadgets and NANOSENSORS geared up with drug delivery abilities can offer sustained drug launch and real time monitoring of drug degrees or biomarkers in the frame.

- Implantable drug delivery systems, which include NANFIBER scaffolds or HYDROGELS, provide ability for long term drug shipping immediately to target tissues or reservoirs, including lymph nodes or viral reservoirs.

CHAPTER FIVE: CHALLENGES AND ETHICAL CONSIDERATIONS

BARRIERS TO DEVELOPING A DEFINITIVE CURE

ACCESS TO TREATMENT AND HEALTHCARE DISPARITIES

Access to remedy and healthcare disparities are big demanding situations in the worldwide reaction to HIV/AIDS. While advances in treatment and prevention have stepped forward consequences for plenty people dwelling with HIV, disparities in access to care persist, in particular among marginalized and susceptible populations.

1. Socioeconomic Factors:

- Socioeconomic fame plays a critical function in get right of entry to to HIV/AIDS remedy and care. Individuals with lower earnings ranges or living in poverty may additionally face boundaries such as lack of medical insurance, restricted access to healthcare centers, and inability to have the funds for medicine and associated fees.

- Economic disparities additionally intersect with different social determinants of fitness, such as race, ethnicity, gender identity, sexual orientation, and geographic place, further exacerbating disparities in get entry to care.

2. Geographic Disparities:

- Access to HIV/AIDS remedy and care varies geographically, with disparities observed among city and rural areas, as well as across exceptional areas and nations.
- Rural and far flung communities can also have restrained healthcare infrastructure, fewer healthcare providers, and demanding situations in having access to specialized HIV/AIDS offerings, such as trying out, remedy, and aid services.

3. Stigma and Discrimination:

- Stigma associated with HIV/AIDS remains a substantial barrier to having access to remedy and care. Fear of discrimination, social ostracism, and violence can deter people from searching for HIV testing, remedy, and help offerings.

- Stigma can be mainly pronounced among positive populations, together with guys who have sex with men.

4. Legal and Policy Barriers:

- Legal and coverage barriers, along with criminalization of HIV transmission, punitive legal guidelines targeting marginalized populations, and restrictive immigration guidelines, can impede get right of entry to HIV/AIDS services and exacerbate fitness disparities.

- Discriminatory legal guidelines and policies might also deter individuals from accessing HIV checking out and remedy or lead to avoidance of healthcare services because of worry of felony repercussions.

5. Healthcare System Challenges:

- Weak healthcare systems, inadequate funding, and healthcare group of workers shortages contribute to disparities in get entry to HIV/AIDS services.

- Healthcare structures may lack vital sources, along with trained healthcare companies, laboratory infrastructure, diagnostic gear, and essential medicinal drugs, restricting the supply and first-rate of HIV/AIDS care.

6. Intersectional Disparities:

INTERSECTIONALITY—the intersecting effect of a couple of sorts of discrimination and drawback—shapes disparities in get entry to HIV/AIDS care. Individuals dealing with multiple marginalized identities, consisting of racial and sexual minorities or transgender people residing in poverty, can also experience compounded obstacles to care.

ADDRESSING GET ENTRY TO DISPARITIES IN HIV/AIDS

- Treatment and care requires complete techniques that address social, financial, structural, and coverage barriers. These strategies may additionally include:

- Expanding access to affordable healthcare services, including HIV testing, treatment, and prevention options.

- Implementing community based approaches that prioritize the needs and perspectives of marginalized populations.

- Advocating for policy changes to address discriminatory laws, reduce stigma, and promote human rights based approaches to HIV/AIDS.

- Strengthening healthcare systems and infrastructure to ensure equitable access to essential HIV/AIDS services for all individuals, regardless of socioeconomic status, geographic location, or identity.

ETHICAL IMPLICATIONS OF GENE EDITING AND OTHER EMERGING TECHNOLOGIES

The emergence of gene enhancing and other superior biotechnologies, together with CRISPRCas9, raises profound ethical implications that necessitate careful attention and deliberation.

1. Informed Consent:

- Ethical issues arise regarding the informed consent process for individuals taking part in gene modifying studies or scientific trials. Participants have to be absolutely knowledgeable about the potential dangers, blessings, and uncertainties related to gene enhancing, in addition to the consequences for themselves and future generations.

2. Safety and Risk Assessment:

- Gene modifying technology has the potential to introduce unintended genetic changes or off target effects, raising worries about safety and long term risks. Ethical pointers and regulatory oversight are needed to make sure rigorous safety assessments and reduce potential damage to research participants and patients.

3. Equitable Access and Justice:

- Ensuring equitable gets right of entry to gene editing remedies and emerging biotechnologies is critical to sell distributive justice and prevent exacerbation of current health disparities. Ethical considerations encompass affordability, accessibility, and prioritization of assets to cope with unmet clinical desires and public fitness priorities.

4. GERMLINE Editing and Heritable Changes:

- GERMLINE modifying, which involves modifying the genetic fabric of embryos, sperm, or eggs, raises ethical concerns approximately heritable changes and the capability effect on future generations. Questions stand up regarding the ethical permissibility, safety, and unintended effects of GERMLINE modifying, including concerns about eugenics, genetic enhancement, and the "slippery slope" towards designer babies.

5. Respect for Human Dignity and Autonomy:

- Ethical principles of appreciate for human dignity, autonomy, and man or woman rights are principal to gene enhancing and biotechnology studies. Respectful and inclusive engagement with diverse stakeholders, consisting of patients, communities, and affected populations, is essential to uphold those concepts and make certain that research and programs align with societal values and norms.

6. Dual Use and Misuse Concerns:

- Gene modifying technologies have DUAL USE capability that means they may be used for each useful and harmful function. Ethical concerns encompass worries approximately bioterrorism, WEAPONIZATION, and unintentional effects of gene enhancing studies, necessitating accountable oversight, transparency, and adherence to BIOSECURITY norms.

7. Environmental and Ecological Implications:

- Gene editing technologies, specifically those concerning genetically modified organisms (GMOs), improve moral questions on environmental effect, ecological sustainability, and unintended outcomes for ecosystems and biodiversity. Ethical frameworks should bear in mind the wider ecological implications of gene enhancing and biotechnology applications.

8. Cultural and Religious Perspectives:

- Ethical views on gene modifying and emerging biotechnologies vary throughout cultural, religious, and philosophical traditions. Ethical deliberations have to be together with diverse viewpoints and values, fostering communicate, mutual recognize, and consensus building amongst stakeholders with unique perspectives.

CHAPTER SIX: GLOBAL COLLABORATION

THE IMPORTANCE OF INTERNATIONAL COOPERATION IN HIV RESEARCH

Joint efforts by using governments, NGOs, and personal sectors

Collaboration among governments, nongovernmental organizations (NGOs), and the private region is vital for addressing complicated worldwide demanding situations which include HIV/AIDS

1. Funding and Resource Mobilization:

- Governments, NGOs, and the personal zone collaborate to mobilize investment and assets for HIV/AIDS prevention, remedy, and research. Initiatives consisting of the Global Fund to Fight AIDS, Tuberculosis, and Malaria depend upon contributions from governments, philanthropic groups, and personal region companions to aid HIV/AIDS packages global.

2. Policy Development and Advocacy:

- Governments, NGOs, and the private sector paintings collectively to broaden evidence based rules, techniques, and advocacy campaigns to cope with HIV/AIDS. This includes advocating for increased investment, strengthening health structures, promoting human rights, and addressing stigma and discrimination associated with HIV/AIDS.

3. Healthcare Delivery and Service Provision:

- Governments collaborate with NGOs and the private sector to supply HIV/AIDS services, consisting of testing, treatment, care, and assist. NGOs frequently play a vital role in offering community based services, outreach applications, and aid for key populations disproportionately affected by HIV/AIDS, which includes guys who've intercourse with men, intercourse workers, those who inject capsules, and transgender individuals.

4. Research and Innovation:

- Governments, NGOs, and the non-public area accomplice to aid HIV/AIDS studies and innovation. This includes funding research, medical trials, and scientific collaborations to develop new treatments, prevention methods, and technologies for HIV/AIDS.

- Public private partnerships (PPPs) facilitate collaboration among authorities agency

5. Capacity Building and Technical Assistance:

- Governments, NGOs, and the private zone collaborate to construct the capability of healthcare employees, researchers, and network corporations to save you, diagnose, and deal with HIV/AIDS. This includes offering education, technical assistance, and mentorship packages to bolster health structures, enhance service delivery, and empower nearby groups.

6. Community Engagement and Participation:

- Governments, NGOs, and the non-public zone interact with affected communities to make sure their meaningful participation in HIV/AIDS applications and decision making strategies. This includes related to humans residing with HIV/AIDS, key populations, and civil society groups in application making plans, implementation, tracking, and assessment.

7. Technology Transfer and Access to Medicines:

- Governments, NGOs, and the private zone collaborate to facilitate generation switch and improve get right of entry to affordable HIV/AIDS drug treatments and technology, especially in low and middle income nations. Initiatives such as voluntary licensing agreements, everyday drug production, and generation transfer partnerships intention to boom get right of entry to critical medicines and reduce remedy costs.

THE ROLE OF ADVOCACY IN RAISING AWARENESS AND FUNDING

Advocacy plays a vital role in raising recognition and funding for HIV/AIDS prevention, remedy, and research.

1. Raising Awareness:

- Advocacy efforts increase public popularity approximately the effect of HIV/AIDS on human beings, organizations, and societies. By disseminating accurate data and hard myths and misconceptions, advocates educate the overall public about the significance of HIV/AIDS prevention, attempting out, and remedy. Advocacy campaigns use diverse channels, consisting of media, social media, community activities, and academic packages, to attain diverse audiences and promote HIV/AIDS focus and information.

2. Reducing Stigma and Discrimination:

- Advocacy campaigns goal to combat stigma and discrimination related to HIV/AIDS, which could deter individuals from searching for checking out, remedy, and aid services. By tough stereotypes, promoting empathy, and fostering inclusive attitudes, advocate's paintings to create environments that are supportive and nonjudgmental for people dwelling with HIV/AIDS.

- Advocacy efforts also deal with structural barriers, which includes discriminatory legal guidelines and rules that perpetuate stigma and undermine get entry to HIV/AIDS services.

3. Empowering Communities:

- Advocacy empowers affected groups, along with humans dwelling with HIV/AIDS, key populations, and marginalized corporations, to suggest for his or her rights, wishes, and priorities. By amplifying their voices and advocating for meaningful participation in decision making processes, advocates make certain that HIV/AIDS responses are inclusive, responsive, and responsible to the ones most affected.

- Community led advocacy projects construct social concord, resilience, and unity, strengthening the ability of communities to mobilize resources, implement programs, and pressure trade at local, countrywide, and worldwide degrees.

4. Shaping Policy and Legislation:

- Advocacy impacts policy and legislative choices associated with HIV/AIDS, shaping the legal and regulatory environment for HIV/AIDS prevention, treatment, and care. Advocates propose for policies that protect human rights, promote get right of entry to services, and cope with underlying social determinants of health.

- Advocacy campaigns mobilize public assist, interact with policymakers, and advocate for evidence based regulations that assist HIV/AIDS prevention, remedy, and studies. Advocates also screen implementation, examine progress, and advocate for coverage reforms whilst wished.

CHAPTER SEVEN: PERSONAL STORIES

NARRATIVES OF INDIVIDUALS LIVING WITH HIV

Testimonials from researchers and scientists on the frontline

Testimonials from researchers and scientists on the frontline of HIV/AIDS studies and response provide treasured insights into the demanding situations, development, and impact in their paintings.

1. Dr. Maria Hernandez, Infectious Disease Researcher:

- "As an infectious disease researcher, I've committed my profession to understanding the complexities of HIV/AIDS and growing progressive strategies for prevention and treatment. Every day, I'm stimulated via the resilience of individuals living with HIV and stimulated to find solutions that improve their great of lifestyles. Collaborating with colleagues and communities, we're making strides in HIV/AIDS research, but there's still a whole lot paintings to be completed to gain our intention of ending the epidemic."

2. Dr. John Smith, Clinical Trials Investigator:

- "Leading clinical trials for brand new HIV/AIDS treatments is each difficult and profitable. It's humbling to witness the impact of innovative remedies on sufferers' lives and to make contributions to the development of scientific technological know-how. However, ensuring get entry to scientific trials and addressing disparities in participation stay crucial priorities. By engaging diverse populations and fostering accept as true with in studies, we will boost up development towards locating a remedy for HIV/AIDS."

3. Dr. Sarah Patel, Public Health Epidemiologist:

- "As a public fitness epidemiologist, my recognition is on knowledge the epidemiology of HIV/AIDS and enforcing evidence based interventions to prevent transmission and enhance health results. Collaborating with groups, policymakers, and healthcare providers, we're working to address the social determinants of health that make contributions to HIV/AIDS disparities. By advocating for equitable get entry to care and addressing stigma and discrimination, we are able to create a extra simply and inclusive society for all."

4. Dr. Carlos Ramirez, Virologist and Vaccine Developer:

- "Developing a powerful HIV vaccine is one of the best demanding situations in biomedical research. Despite Stories of hope and resilience in the face of the epidemic

Stories of hope and resilience within the face of the HIV/AIDS epidemic spotlight the power and courage of people, groups, and businesses suffering from the sickness.

1. The Lazarus Effect:

- The "Lazarus effect" refers back to the wonderful recovery of individuals dwelling with HIV/AIDS who enjoy a dramatic improvement in fitness and wellbeing after receiving antiretroviral treatment (ART). For many humans, ART transforms HIV/AIDS from a life threatening infection to a attainable persistent circumstance, allowing them to lead wholesome and efficient lives.
- These memories of "resurrection" symbolize the transformative energy of get admission to treatment and care,

presenting hope to tens of millions of people living with HIV/AIDS round the sector.

2. Community Support and Solidarity:

- Many groups tormented by HIV/AIDS have come together to provide mutual assist, harmony, and compassion to those residing with the disorder. Community based groups, guide corporations, and peer networks offer emotional guide, sensible help, and advocacy for people and households suffering from HIV/AIDS.

- These stories of network resilience demonstrate the electricity of collective action and cohesion in addressing the social, financial, and mental challenges of residing with HIV/AIDS.

3. Advocacy and Activism:

- HIV/AIDS advocacy and activism have played a pivotal role in elevating attention, difficult stigma, and advocating for the rights and dignity of people residing with HIV/AIDS. Activists, advocates, and allies have fought tirelessly forget admission to remedy, healthcare, and social justice for all individuals tormented by HIV/AIDS.

- These tales of advocacy and activism spotlight the courage and backbone of people and groups who have mobilized communities,

- These stories of personal resilience and triumph demonstrate the human capacity to overcome obstacles, find strength in adversity, and embrace life with courage and optimism.

CHAPTER EIGHT: FUTURE PROSPECTS

THE POTENTIAL TIMELINE FOR A CURE

Addressing ongoing challenges in HIV prevention and treatment

Addressing ongoing demanding situations in HIV prevention and remedy calls for complete techniques that address the complex interaction of biomedical, behavioral, social, and structural factors contributing to the HIV/AIDS epidemic.

1. Stigma and Discrimination:

- Challenge: Stigma and discrimination continue to be substantial obstacles to HIV prevention, checking out, and treatment, leading to worry, secrecy, and reluctance to seek services among affected populations.

- Approach: Addressing stigma and discrimination calls for multilevel interventions that sell consciousness, project stereotypes, and foster inclusive and supportive environments for people dwelling with HIV/AIDS. Community based programs, media campaigns, and advocacy efforts can help lessen stigma and promote attractiveness and empathy.

2. Access to Testing and Treatment:

- Challenge: Limited get right of entry to HIV trying out and remedy services, especially in marginalized and underserved groups, impedes efforts to diagnose and deal with HIV/AIDS early and successfully.

- Approach: Strengthening healthcare structures, expanding get entry to HIV trying out and remedy services, and integrating HIV services into existing healthcare infrastructure are important. Innovative approaches which include community based testing, mobile clinics, and self testing kits can improve get

admission to and reach underserved
populations.

3. Prevention Strategies for Key Populations:

- Challenge: Key populations
  disproportionately tormented by
  HIV/AIDS, which include guys who have
  sex with men, transgender individuals, sex
  employees, folks who inject tablets, and
  incarcerated people, face specific
  challenges in having access to HIV
  prevention and remedy offerings.

4. HIV Prevention among Adolescents and Young
People:

- Challenge: Adolescents and younger
  human beings are disproportionately
  affected by HIV/AIDS, yet face
  limitations together with restricted get
  entry to complete sexuality schooling,
  healthcare offerings, and HIV prevention
  interventions.

- Approach: Implementing complete sexuality education programs in faculties, youth friendly healthcare offerings, and centered HIV prevention interventions for younger humans can help lessen HIV prevalence and empower youngsters to make knowledgeable selections approximately their sexual fitness.

5. Addressing Confections and Co morbidities:

- Challenge: HIV/AIDS is regularly associated with confections, which includes tuberculosis (TB), hepatitis B and C, and no communicable illnesses (NCDs) like cardiovascular disease and diabetes, which complicate remedy and management.

- Approach: Strengthening integrated healthcare offerings that deal with HIV/AIDS, confections, and co morbidities is critical. This consists of screening, prognosis, and remedy for confections, in addition to selling healthful existence and preventive measures to lessen the risk of NCDs amongst human beings dwelling with HIV/AIDS.

6. Ensuring Sustainable Funding and Resources:

- Challenge: Sustainable investment and sources are hard to guide HIV prevention, remedy, and research efforts, yet economic commitments vary and may be insufficient to meet the developing wishes of the HIV/AIDS reaction.

- Approach: Advocating for improved investment in HIV/AIDS programs and research, strengthening health financing structures, and selling domestic aid mobilization are essential. Sustainable financing mechanisms, revolutionary financing models, and partnerships between governments, donors, and the

private quarter can help make certain
long-term sustainability of HIV/AIDS

THE OUTLOOK FOR ERADICATING HIV/AIDS GLOBALLY

Eradicating HIV/AIDS globally remains a complicated and challenging goal, however huge development has been made in recent years, and there are motives for optimism.

1. Advances in Treatment and Prevention:

- The development of effective antiretroviral therapy (ART) has converted HIV/AIDS from a life threatening infection to a potential chronic circumstance for lots humans living with HIV. ART no longer most effective improves health effects and decreases mortality however also reduces the threat of HIV transmission.

- Innovations in HIV prevention strategies, including PREEXPOSURE prophylaxis (PREP), treatment as prevention (TASP), voluntary medical male circumcision (VMMC), and damage discount programs for those who inject capsules, have contributed to declines in HIV prevalence in lots of settings.

2. Global Targets and Commitments:

- The international network has set bold targets for finishing the HIV/AIDS epidemic, together with the UNAIDS 959595 goals with the aid of 2030: 95% of human beings residing with HIV recognize their repute, ninety five% of these recognized acquire ART, and ninety five% of these on remedy obtain viral suppression.

- Countries round the world have committed to those objectives through projects along with the United Nations Sustainable Development Goals (SDGs) and the Global Fund to Fight AIDS, Tuberculosis, and Malaria.

3. Scientific Innovation and Research:

- Scientific advances in HIV/AIDS research, consisting of vaccine improvement, gene modifying technology, and long acting antiretroviral formulations, keep promise for brand new prevention and remedy options.

- Ongoing research efforts are focused on finding a cure for HIV/AIDS, including strategies to eliminate viral reservoirs, enhance immune responses, and eradicate HIV from the body.

4. Community Engagement and Empowerment:

- Community led responses to HIV/AIDS play a vital role in prevention, treatment, and advocacy efforts. Engaging affected communities, inclusive of humans living with HIV/AIDS, key populations, and marginalized businesses, is essential for designing effective interventions, reducing stigma, and promoting access to offerings.

5. Political Commitment and Leadership:

- Political commitment and management at all ranges are vital for riding progress toward ending the HIV/AIDS epidemic. Governments, policymakers, and civil society leaders ought to prioritize HIV/AIDS on political agendas, allocate sources efficiently, and put in force evidence based totally policies and packages.

- Despite those promising tendencies, big challenges remain on the path to removing HIV/AIDS globally:

1. Health Inequities and Disparities:

- Health inequities and disparities in access to HIV/AIDS services persist, especially among marginalized and vulnerable populations. Addressing social determinants of health, reducing stigma and discrimination, and selling health equity are crucial for accomplishing the ones most laid low with HIV/AIDS.

2. Funding and Resource Gaps:

- Funding shortfalls and resource gaps pose challenges to sustaining and scaling up HIV/AIDS programs and offerings. Increased investment, advanced useful resource allocation, and innovative financing mechanisms are hard to make sure the long term sustainability of the HIV/AIDS response.

3. Emerging Challenges:

- Emerging challenges, which includes the effect of the COVID19 pandemic on HIV/AIDS offerings, the upward push of drug resistant lines of HIV, and the persistence of prison and policy limitations, require ongoing attention and revolutionary solutions.

www.ingramcontent.com/pod-product-compliance
Lightning Source LLC
Chambersburg PA
CBHW050844260726
48660CB00006B/2438